The Galveston Diet

Pros & Cons for Perimenopausal Women

CONTENT

Chapter 1:
Introduction to the Galveston Diet

Overview of the Galveston Diet and its Founder, Dr. Mary Claire Haver

The Galveston Diet is a unique and increasingly popular weight loss program designed specifically to address the challenges faced by perimenopausal women. Founded by Dr. Mary Claire Haver, an accomplished obstetrician-gynecologist, this diet plan has gained recognition for its effectiveness in helping women navigate the complexities of weight gain during the perimenopausal phase.

Dr. Mary Claire Haver's journey towards developing the Galveston Diet was deeply rooted in her own personal experience. Like many of her patients, she found herself grappling with the frustrating and often disheartening issue of weight gain as she entered the perimenopausal stage.

Traditional weight loss advice, which often revolves around the simple mantra of "eat less and move more," proved to be largely ineffective for her and her patients. This prompted her to explore a new approach, one that would cater to the unique challenges faced by women during perimenopause.

Dr. Haver's medical background provided her with valuable insights into the intricacies of the female body's hormonal changes during perimenopause. She recognized that these changes, combined with factors such as aging and lifestyle, played a pivotal role in the onset of weight gain during this phase of a woman's life. Driven by a desire to not only understand but also combat this issue, she embarked on a mission to create a diet plan that would address the root causes of perimenopausal weight gain.

The Galveston Diet is the culmination of Dr. Haver's extensive research and expertise in women's health. What sets this program apart is its emphasis on hormonal balance and a holistic approach to weight loss. Dr. Haver's background as an obstetrician-gynecologist provided her with a deep understanding of the female hormonal system, and she applied this knowledge to develop a program tailored specifically to women experiencing perimenopause.

The Galveston Diet is a reflection of Dr. Haver's commitment to helping women not only shed excess weight but also regain control over their bodies during a phase of life that can be challenging both physically and emotionally. With a medical professional at the helm, this program offers a sense of trust and reliability, ensuring that it is founded on scientific principles and expert knowledge.

Explanation of the Perimenopausal Challenges and How This Diet Addresses Them

Perimenopause, often referred to as the menopausal transition, is a natural and inevitable phase in a woman's life. It typically occurs in the late 40s or early 50s but can vary from woman to woman. During this phase, the body undergoes a series of hormonal changes that prepare it for the eventual cessation of menstruation, which marks the onset of menopause.

One of the most significant challenges faced by women during perimenopause is the occurrence of hormonal imbalances. Estrogen and progesterone, two key female hormones, fluctuate erratically, causing a cascade of physiological changes. These hormonal fluctuations can lead to a range of symptoms, including hot flashes, mood swings, disrupted sleep, and, notably, weight gain.

Weight gain during perimenopause is a multifaceted issue. Several factors contribute to this phenomenon:

1. **Slowed Metabolism**: As women age, their metabolism naturally slows down. This means that the body burns calories at a slower rate, making it easier to gain weight, even when calorie intake remains the same.

2. **Hormonal Changes**: The fluctuating levels of estrogen and progesterone can disrupt the body's ability to maintain a healthy weight. These hormonal imbalances often lead to increased fat storage, particularly around the abdomen.

3. **Muscle Loss**: Aging, combined with hormonal changes, can result in a loss of lean muscle mass. Muscle plays a vital role in calorie burning, and its reduction contributes to weight gain.

4. **Changes in Appetite**: Many women experience changes in appetite and food cravings during perimenopause. This can lead to overeating and a preference for unhealthy, calorie-dense foods.

5. **Stress and Sleep Issues**: The hormonal fluctuations in perimenopause can also impact stress levels and sleep patterns. High stress and inadequate sleep can further exacerbate weight gain.

The Galveston Diet addresses these perimenopausal challenges through a comprehensive approach that emphasizes hormonal balance and anti-inflammatory foods. Rather than relying solely on calorie restriction, which often proves ineffective during perimenopause due to a slowed metabolism, Dr. Haver's program focuses on the quality of the foods consumed.

By prioritizing anti-inflammatory whole foods, the Galveston Diet aims to create an environment in which hormones can function optimally. The plan encourages the consumption of lean proteins, fruits, vegetables, legumes, whole grains, healthy fats, and full-fat dairy—all of which support hormonal balance and overall health.

Furthermore, the diet discourages processed foods containing added sugars, artificial ingredients, and inflammatory substances. These items are known to cause inflammation in the body, which can further disrupt hormonal balance and exacerbate weight gain during perimenopause.

In addition to dietary guidelines, the Galveston Diet incorporates intermittent fasting, a strategy that has shown promise in supporting weight loss and hormonal balance. Dr. Haver specifically recommends the 16:8 method, which involves fasting for 16 hours and eating within an 8-hour window. This approach, according to Dr. Haver, not only assists in calorie restriction but also offers neuroprotective and anti-inflammatory benefits.

The Galveston Diet's holistic approach addresses the root causes of perimenopausal weight gain, making it a comprehensive and targeted solution for women facing the challenges of this life stage.

Importance of Hormonal Balance in Weight Loss for Women

Hormonal balance is a critical factor in the journey of weight loss for women, and it takes on even greater significance during perimenopause. The female body's intricate hormonal system plays a substantial role in regulating various physiological functions, including metabolism, appetite, and fat storage.

Hormones such as estrogen and progesterone, which undergo significant fluctuations during perimenopause, directly influence how the body manages weight. Understanding the importance of hormonal balance in weight loss is pivotal to appreciating the Galveston Diet's approach.

Here's why hormonal balance matters:

1. Metabolism Regulation: Hormones, including thyroid hormones, play a crucial role in regulating metabolism—the process by which the body converts food into energy. When hormones are imbalanced, metabolism can slow down, making it harder to burn calories efficiently.

2. Appetite Control: Leptin and ghrelin, often referred to as hunger hormones, help regulate appetite. Hormonal imbalances can disrupt the body's hunger cues, leading to increased appetite and a tendency to overeat.

3. Fat Storage: Estrogen, in particular, influences fat distribution in the body. As estrogen levels fluctuate during perimenopause, women often notice weight gain in the abdominal area, which is associated with increased health risks.

4. Insulin Sensitivity: Hormones also impact insulin sensitivity, which affects how the body processes and stores carbohydrates. Hormonal imbalances can lead to insulin resistance, making it harder to control blood sugar levels and manage weight.

5. Mood and Stress Management: Hormones play a significant role in mood regulation. Imbalances can contribute to mood swings and increased stress, which may lead to emotional eating and weight gain.

In essence, hormonal imbalances can create an environment within the body that promotes weight gain and makes it challenging to shed excess pounds. This is precisely where the Galveston Diet's emphasis on anti-inflammatory foods and intermittent fasting comes into play.

The program's approach revolves around supporting hormonal balance by providing the body with the necessary nutrients and minimizing the intake of foods that promote inflammation. By doing so, it creates an environment in which hormones can function optimally, aiding in weight loss and overall well-being.

Chapter 2: Understanding Menopausal Weight Gain

Menopause is a natural and inevitable phase in a woman's life, signifying the end of her reproductive years. This transition, however, comes with a variety of physical, emotional, and hormonal changes that can significantly impact a woman's body and overall well-being. One of the most common and frustrating issues that women face during this period is weight gain. In this chapter, we will delve into the hormonal changes that occur during menopause, explore the factors contributing to weight gain in perimenopausal women, and understand why traditional weight loss methods often fail during this life stage.

Hormonal Changes During Menopause

Hormones play a pivotal role in regulating various bodily functions, including metabolism, appetite, and fat storage. As women enter perimenopause and eventually reach menopause, their hormonal landscape undergoes significant shifts. These hormonal changes are closely linked to the weight gain experienced during this life stage.

Estrogen Decline

Estrogen is a primary female sex hormone that is produced by the ovaries. During perimenopause, which can start in a woman's late 30s or early 40s, estrogen production begins to decline. This decline becomes more pronounced as menopause approaches. Estrogen is not only responsible for the regulation of the menstrual cycle but also has a profound impact on how the body stores and uses fat. As estrogen levels drop, it can lead to an increase in fat accumulation, especially around the abdominal area.

The reduction in estrogen levels also affects the body's ability to respond to insulin, which can result in insulin resistance. Insulin resistance makes it more challenging for the body to regulate blood sugar levels and can lead to increased fat storage, particularly in the abdominal region. This phenomenon can contribute to the development of metabolic syndrome, a cluster of conditions that increase the risk of heart disease, stroke, and type 2 diabetes.

Progesterone Imbalance

In addition to estrogen decline, perimenopausal women often experience imbalances in progesterone, another important hormone. Progesterone plays a role in maintaining a healthy weight by promoting the use of fat for energy and balancing estrogen's effects. As progesterone levels decrease, this delicate hormonal balance is disrupted, which can result in weight gain.

Thyroid Function

Thyroid hormones also play a crucial role in regulating metabolism and energy expenditure. Many perimenopausal women may experience changes in thyroid function, leading to a slowing of metabolism. This decrease in metabolic rate can make it more challenging to maintain or lose weight.

Leptin and Ghrelin

Leptin and ghrelin are hormones that regulate appetite and satiety. Leptin, produced by fat cells, sends signals to the brain to reduce hunger and increase energy expenditure. Ghrelin, produced in the stomach, stimulates appetite. During menopause, hormonal imbalances can disrupt the communication between these hormones, leading to increased hunger and decreased feelings of fullness. This can result in overeating and weight gain.

Factors Contributing to Weight Gain in Perimenopausal Women

Several factors contribute to weight gain during perimenopause and menopause, often interacting with the hormonal changes discussed above. Understanding these factors is essential for addressing weight gain effectively.

Muscle Loss

As women age, they naturally lose muscle mass. With decreased muscle mass, the body's ability to burn calories diminishes. This loss of muscle tissue can be accelerated during menopause, making it more challenging to maintain a healthy weight.

Lifestyle Changes

The perimenopausal phase often coincides with significant lifestyle changes. Many women in this age group are dealing with increased work responsibilities, caring for children, and even aging parents. These demands can lead to stress and decreased physical activity, both of which contribute to weight gain.

Dietary Habits

Changes in dietary habits can also contribute to weight gain. Some women may consume more calories as a way to cope with the emotional and physical challenges of menopause. Additionally, the consumption of processed and high-sugar foods can lead to weight gain and exacerbate hormonal imbalances.

Stress and Sleep

Stress and sleep play a crucial role in hormonal balance and weight regulation. High levels of stress can lead to increased cortisol production, a hormone associated with abdominal fat storage. Poor sleep quality, which is common during menopause, can disrupt the body's ability to regulate hormones related to hunger and appetite, leading to overeating.

Genetics

Genetics also play a role in how women experience weight gain during menopause. Some women may be genetically predisposed to accumulate fat around the abdomen, making it even more challenging to maintain a healthy weight.

Why Traditional Weight Loss Methods Often Fail

Traditional weight loss methods that rely solely on calorie restriction and increased physical activity often fall short in addressing the unique challenges faced by perimenopausal and menopausal women. Here are several reasons why these methods may be less effective during this life stage:

Hormonal Imbalances

Traditional weight loss methods do not account for the hormonal changes that are occurring. Calorie restriction without addressing hormonal balance can lead to muscle loss and slowed metabolism, exacerbating the problem.

Metabolic Rate

As mentioned earlier, the decrease in metabolic rate during menopause can make it difficult for women to lose weight through conventional methods. Simply cutting calories without addressing the underlying metabolic changes may result in minimal weight loss.

Psychological Factors

Menopause is a time of emotional and psychological change as well. Traditional diets often overlook the emotional aspects of eating. Emotional eating, stress, and poor body image can make it challenging to adhere to a strict diet and exercise plan.

Sustainability

Many traditional weight loss methods are difficult to sustain in the long term. Perimenopausal and menopausal women need approaches that are not only effective but also practical and sustainable for the rest of their lives.

Chapter 3:
The Science Behind the Galveston Diet

In this chapter, we will delve into the science underpinning the Galveston Diet, focusing on two critical aspects: the role of anti-inflammatory foods in hormonal balance and the concept of intermittent fasting and its effects on the body. We will also review relevant research that supports these key components of the diet.

The Role of Anti-Inflammatory Foods in Hormonal Balance

Hormones play a pivotal role in regulating various physiological processes within the body, including metabolism, appetite, and fat storage. For women, hormonal imbalances, particularly during perimenopause and menopause, can lead to weight gain and a host of other health issues. The Galveston Diet acknowledges this and places a strong emphasis on anti-inflammatory foods to help restore hormonal balance. Let's explore this in detail:

1. Understanding Inflammation:

- Inflammation is the body's natural response to injury or infection. However, chronic inflammation can disrupt hormonal balance and contribute to weight gain.

- Pro-inflammatory foods, such as those high in sugar, refined carbohydrates, and unhealthy fats, can exacerbate inflammation and hormone-related problems.

2. Anti-Inflammatory Foods:

- The Galveston Diet encourages the consumption of anti-inflammatory foods that help reduce chronic inflammation. These include:

  - Fruits and vegetables: Rich in antioxidants, vitamins, and minerals, they combat oxidative stress and reduce inflammation.

  - Fatty fish: Sources of omega-3 fatty acids, which have potent anti-inflammatory properties.

  - Nuts and seeds: Provide healthy fats and antioxidants that support hormonal health.

- Whole grains: High in fiber, they stabilize blood sugar levels and reduce inflammation.

- Full-fat dairy: Contains conjugated linoleic acid (CLA) and helps in hormonal regulation.

3. Hormone Regulation:

- By consuming these anti-inflammatory foods, the Galveston Diet aims to regulate hormones such as insulin, cortisol, and leptin, which play crucial roles in metabolism, appetite, and fat storage.

- Hormone regulation helps women achieve and maintain a healthy weight, even during perimenopause when hormonal fluctuations can lead to stubborn fat gain.

4. Avoiding Inflammatory Foods:

- In addition to promoting anti-inflammatory foods, the Galveston Diet advises against consuming pro-inflammatory foods. This means avoiding or minimizing processed foods, added sugars, artificial ingredients, and unhealthy fats.

By prioritizing anti-inflammatory foods and reducing inflammation in the body, the Galveston Diet aims to restore hormonal balance, making it easier for perimenopausal women to lose weight and maintain a healthy lifestyle.

Explaining the Concept of Intermittent Fasting and Its Effects on the Body

Intermittent fasting (IF) is a fundamental component of the Galveston Diet, and it's essential to understand how it works and its effects on the body. Intermittent fasting is not just about calorie restriction; it brings about specific changes in the body that support weight loss and overall health. Let's explore this concept:

1. What Is Intermittent Fasting?

- Intermittent fasting is an eating pattern that alternates between periods of eating and fasting.

- The Galveston Diet primarily recommends the 16:8 method, where individuals fast for 16 hours and eat during an 8-hour window. This approach is known for its simplicity and effectiveness.

2. Hormonal Changes:

- Intermittent fasting triggers hormonal changes that promote fat loss. These changes include increased levels of:

    - Human Growth Hormone (HGH): HGH helps with fat breakdown and muscle preservation.

    - Norepinephrine: This hormone boosts metabolism and encourages fat release from fat cells.

    - Insulin Sensitivity: IF enhances insulin sensitivity, reducing the risk of insulin resistance and diabetes.

3. Autophagy:

- Intermittent fasting induces a process called autophagy, which is the body's way of cleaning out damaged cells and regenerating new, healthy ones. This process is linked to improved longevity and cellular health.

4. Caloric Restriction vs. Intermittent Fasting:

- While both caloric restriction and intermittent fasting lead to weight loss, the latter offers unique benefits beyond simple calorie reduction.

- Research suggests that intermittent fasting may be more sustainable and easier to adhere to than continuous caloric restriction.

5. 16:8 Method vs. 5:2 Method:

- The Galveston Diet recommends the 16:8 method over the 5:2 method (eating 500 calories for two days per week).

- Dr. Haver argues that the 16:8 method is more practical for most people and aligns well with hormonal balance.

Reviewing Relevant Research on Anti-Inflammatory Diets and Intermittent Fasting

1. Anti-Inflammatory Diets:

- Numerous studies have shown the benefits of anti-inflammatory diets in reducing inflammation and improving hormonal balance.

- Research supports the role of antioxidants, omega-3 fatty acids, and fiber in mitigating inflammation.

- These diets are linked to weight loss and better metabolic health.

2. Intermittent Fasting:

- Research on intermittent fasting has demonstrated its effectiveness in weight loss and metabolic improvements.

- Studies indicate that intermittent fasting may offer unique advantages over continuous caloric restriction.

- It's essential to note that more research is ongoing, particularly regarding long-term effects and individual suitability.

Chapter 4:
What You Can Eat on the Galveston Diet

In this chapter, we will delve into the specifics of the Galveston Diet, outlining the comprehensive list of allowed foods, providing sample meal plans and recipes that emphasize anti-inflammatory ingredients, and offering practical tips for meal preparation and planning.

Comprehensive List of Allowed Foods

The Galveston Diet places a strong emphasis on consuming anti-inflammatory foods, as these are believed to play a crucial role in helping perimenopausal women achieve hormonal balance and combat weight gain. Here's a breakdown of the key food categories that are encouraged on this diet:

1. Whole Grains:

- Whole grains, such as quinoa, brown rice, and whole wheat, are rich in fiber and essential nutrients. They provide sustained energy and help regulate blood sugar levels, which can be especially beneficial for women experiencing hormonal fluctuations.

2. Lean Proteins:

- Lean protein sources like skinless poultry, fish, and lean cuts of meat are central to the Galveston Diet. Protein is essential for muscle preservation and satiety, and it helps prevent muscle loss during weight loss efforts.

3. Fruits:

- Fruits are a natural source of vitamins, minerals, and antioxidants. Berries, citrus fruits, and apples are particularly recommended due to their anti-inflammatory properties. They also provide a touch of sweetness to meals and snacks without the need for added sugars.

4. Vegetables:

- A wide variety of vegetables is encouraged, especially those that are colorful and packed with nutrients. Spinach, kale, broccoli, and sweet potatoes are some of the top choices. These vegetables are loaded with antioxidants, vitamins, and minerals that support overall health.

5. Legumes:

- Legumes, such as lentils, chickpeas, and black beans, are excellent sources of plant-based protein and fiber. They help with appetite control and provide essential nutrients that promote hormone balance.

6. Healthy Fats:

- Healthy fats, including olive oil, fatty fish (like salmon), and nuts and seeds, are crucial for hormone production and overall well-being. Omega-3 fatty acids, found in fatty fish and certain nuts and seeds, have anti-inflammatory properties that can aid in hormonal regulation.

7. Full-Fat Dairy:

- Contrary to some popular beliefs, full-fat dairy is allowed on the Galveston Diet. Full-fat dairy products, such as yogurt and cheese, provide essential nutrients like calcium and vitamin D. They can also contribute to a feeling of fullness, reducing the likelihood of overeating.

It's important to note that while these food categories are encouraged, processed foods, added sugars, artificial ingredients, and inflammatory oils should be limited or avoided. These restrictions align with the anti-inflammatory nature of the diet, which aims to reduce inflammation and support hormone balance.

Sample Meal Plans and Recipes Emphasizing Anti-Inflammatory Ingredients

To help you get started with the Galveston Diet, let's explore some sample meal plans and recipes that showcase the principles of this approach.

Sample Breakfast Meal Plan:

- **Breakfast:** Greek yogurt parfait with mixed berries and a sprinkle of chopped nuts.

- **Morning Snack:** Sliced cucumber and carrot sticks with hummus.

- **Lunch:** Quinoa and roasted vegetable salad with grilled chicken.

- **Afternoon Snack:** A piece of whole fruit, like an apple or an orange.

- **Dinner:** Baked salmon with a side of steamed broccoli and quinoa.

- **Dessert:** A small serving of dark chocolate.

These meal plans and recipes illustrate the Galveston Diet's focus on whole, nutrient-dense foods that support hormone balance and combat inflammation.

Tips for Meal Preparation and Planning

Successful adherence to the Galveston Diet often involves thoughtful meal preparation and planning. Here are some practical tips to help you incorporate this dietary approach into your lifestyle:

1. **Meal Prep:** Dedicate some time each week to prepare staples like quinoa, lean protein, and chopped vegetables. Having these components ready makes assembling meals quick and convenient.

2. **Variety:** Rotate your food choices to ensure you get a wide range of nutrients. Experiment with different fruits, vegetables, and grains to keep your meals interesting.

3. **Portion Control:** While whole, anti-inflammatory foods are encouraged, portion control is still essential for weight management. Be mindful of portion sizes to avoid overeating.

4. **Hydration:** Don't forget the importance of staying hydrated. Water and herbal teas can aid digestion and overall well-being.

5. **Seek Support:** Consider sharing your journey with a friend or family member. Having a support system can make it easier to stick to your dietary goals.

6. **Consult a Dietitian:** If you have specific dietary concerns or questions, consulting a registered dietitian can provide personalized guidance tailored to your unique needs and goals.

Incorporating these tips into your daily routine can help you make the most of the Galveston Diet and potentially find success in your weight loss and hormonal balance journey.

Chapter 5:
The 16:8 Intermittent Fasting Method

Intermittent fasting (IF) has gained popularity in recent years as a weight loss and health strategy. One specific approach, the 16:8 fasting method, is a central component of the Galveston Diet designed to combat menopausal weight gain. In this chapter, we will delve into the details of the 16:8 fasting method, explore its benefits, address common concerns and misconceptions, and share inspiring testimonials from women who have experienced success with this approach.

Explanation of the 16:8 Fasting Method and Its Benefits

What Is the 16:8 Fasting Method?

The 16:8 fasting method, also known as time-restricted eating, is a type of intermittent fasting that involves cycling between periods of eating and fasting. The name "16:8" comes from the fasting and eating windows within a 24-hour day. During the 16:8 method, you fast for 16 hours and restrict your eating to an 8-hour window.

How Does It Work?

- Fasting Window: This method typically involves fasting from the evening until the next day, allowing you to skip breakfast and delay your first meal until later in the day.

- Eating Window: You consume your daily caloric intake within the 8-hour eating window, which often begins in the late morning or early afternoon.

Benefits of the 16:8 Fasting Method

The 16:8 fasting method offers several potential benefits, which may explain its appeal and inclusion in the Galveston Diet:

1. **Weight Loss:** By limiting the time available for eating, the 16:8 method naturally reduces your daily calorie intake, which can lead to weight loss. However, it's important to note that any calorie restriction can result in weight loss, so the 16:8 method is not a magical solution but rather a structured way to control calorie intake.

2. **Improved Hormonal Balance:** One of the unique aspects of the 16:8 method is its potential to support hormonal balance. Fasting periods may enhance insulin sensitivity and reduce insulin resistance, which is particularly beneficial for women dealing with hormonal fluctuations during perimenopause.

3. **Enhanced Fat Burning:** During the fasting window, your body primarily relies on stored fat for energy since you're not consuming new calories. This promotes fat loss and can be particularly effective for stubborn areas of fat that tend to accumulate during menopause.

4. **Simplicity and Sustainability:** The 16:8 method is relatively straightforward and doesn't involve complex calorie counting or macronutrient tracking. This simplicity makes it a more sustainable approach for many individuals, as it can easily fit into daily routines.

5. **Reduction in Snacking:** Having a defined eating window can help curb mindless snacking, which is a

common contributor to weight gain. Knowing that you have a specific time to eat encourages mindfulness about food choices.

Addressing Common Concerns and Misconceptions about Intermittent Fasting

1. Concern: Fasting Will Slow Down Metabolism

Misconception: Many people fear that fasting may slow down their metabolism, leading to reduced energy expenditure and potential weight gain.

Reality: Research on intermittent fasting, including the 16:8 method, suggests that it does not significantly affect basal metabolic rate. In fact, it can enhance fat oxidation and promote weight loss when combined with a balanced diet.

2. Concern: Skipping Breakfast Is Unhealthy

Misconception: Breakfast is often touted as the most important meal of the day, and skipping it is believed to be detrimental to health.

Reality: The 16:8 method doesn't necessarily mean skipping breakfast; it merely shifts your first meal to a later time. Research shows that the timing of meals may not be as critical as the quality and quantity of food consumed. What matters is that you maintain a balanced diet within your eating window.

3. Concern: Fasting Leads to Muscle Loss

Misconception: Fasting for extended periods may lead to muscle loss, causing a decrease in overall strength and physical fitness.

Reality: When done correctly, intermittent fasting, including the 16:8 method, can help preserve lean muscle mass while promoting fat loss. Adequate protein intake during the eating window is crucial for maintaining muscle.

4. Concern: Intermittent Fasting Is Only for Certain Groups

Misconception: Intermittent fasting is suitable for only specific groups of people and may not be safe for everyone.

Reality: While intermittent fasting is generally safe and effective, it may not be suitable for individuals with specific medical conditions or those taking certain medications. It's essential to consult a healthcare professional before starting any fasting regimen, especially if you have diabetes or a history of eating disorders.

Testimonials and Success Stories from Women Who Have Tried the 16:8 Method

Real-life experiences and success stories can be highly motivating for individuals considering the 16:8 fasting method. Let's hear from women who have embraced this approach and achieved positive results:

Testimonial 1: Jane's Journey to Menopausal Weight Loss

Jane, a 52-year-old woman struggling with perimenopausal weight gain, decided to give the 16:8 method a try after reading about it in the Galveston Diet program. She shares, "The 16:8 method was a game-changer for me. It allowed me to regain control over my eating habits and shed those stubborn pounds that seemed impossible to lose. Plus, I noticed improved energy levels and better sleep, which were unexpected bonuses."

Testimonial 2: Sarah's Hormonal Balance

Sarah, 48, faced hormonal imbalances that were exacerbating her menopausal weight gain. She says, "Intermittent fasting helped me balance my hormones, especially insulin. I saw a significant reduction in my sugar cravings, which made it easier to stick to a healthier diet.

The 16:8 method became a sustainable part of my life, and I'm no longer a slave to the scale."

Testimonial 3: Maria's Health Transformation

Maria, a 55-year-old woman, tried the 16:8 method not just for weight loss but for overall health improvements. She reflects, "Intermittent fasting helped me gain clarity about my eating patterns and taught me to distinguish between true hunger and emotional eating. It's not just about the weight I've lost; it's about the freedom I've gained from food cravings and emotional eating triggers."

Chapter 6:
Pros and Cons of the Galveston Diet

In this chapter, we'll take an in-depth look at the pros and cons of the Galveston Diet, a weight loss program designed for perimenopausal women. Understanding both the benefits and drawbacks of this diet will help you make an informed decision about whether it's the right choice for you.

Pros of the Galveston Diet

Sustainable Approach

One of the standout features of the Galveston Diet is its sustainable approach to weight loss. Unlike many fad diets that require extreme restrictions or quick fixes, this program emphasizes a long-term, manageable lifestyle change. Rather than obsessing over calorie counting or strict macronutrient ratios, the Galveston Diet encourages you to focus on the quality of the foods you consume.

The sustainable aspect of this diet is especially appealing to perimenopausal women who may have tried various diets in the past, only to find that they were difficult to maintain. By shifting the focus to anti-inflammatory foods and whole, nutritious ingredients, the Galveston Diet offers a more practical and enjoyable way to approach weight loss. It's not about deprivation but about nourishing your body with foods that promote hormonal balance and overall well-being.

Emphasis on Whole Foods

The Galveston Diet places a strong emphasis on whole foods. It encourages the consumption of lean proteins, fruits, vegetables, legumes, whole grains, healthy fats, and full-fat dairy products. This focus on unprocessed, natural foods provides a multitude of health benefits.

Whole foods are rich in vitamins, minerals, and antioxidants, all of which play essential roles in maintaining good health. They are also less likely to cause inflammation in the body, making them ideal choices for perimenopausal women looking to combat weight gain. By including a variety of whole foods in your diet, you're not only working toward weight loss but also promoting overall wellness.

Hormone Balance

The primary goal of the Galveston Diet is to address the hormonal imbalances that often occur during perimenopause, which can lead to weight gain. Dr. Mary Claire Haver, the creator of the diet, recognized that simply reducing calories or increasing physical activity was not sufficient to tackle this issue. Instead, the program focuses on the vital role that anti-inflammatory foods play in hormonal balance.

Many foods included in the diet, such as fatty fish, nuts, and seeds, contain essential fatty acids that can help regulate hormones. Additionally, the diet's emphasis on whole foods provides a steady source of nutrients that support overall hormonal health.

By promoting hormone balance through nutrition, the Galveston Diet seeks to help women in perimenopause manage their weight more effectively than traditional dieting methods.

Cons of the Galveston Diet

Lack of Specific Research

One significant drawback of the Galveston Diet is the lack of specific scientific research directly supporting its effectiveness. While the diet's principles, such as consuming anti-inflammatory foods and practicing intermittent fasting, are rooted in existing scientific knowledge, there is no dedicated research on this particular program.

This absence of data leaves some uncertainty about the diet's outcomes, including its long-term impact on weight loss and health. Without studies specific to the Galveston Diet, it's challenging to gauge the extent of its success or whether it's the best approach for every perimenopausal woman.

Limitations of Intermittent Fasting

Intermittent fasting is a cornerstone of the Galveston Diet. While many people have experienced success with this approach, it's important to note that intermittent fasting may not be suitable for everyone. Dr. Haver recommends the 16:8 method, where you fast for 16 hours and eat during an 8-hour window. However, it's crucial to consider individual circumstances and preferences.

Some individuals, such as those with diabetes, certain medical conditions, or a history of eating disorders, may not find intermittent fasting to be the best option. Additionally, some people may struggle with the strict time restrictions imposed by fasting, and it could lead to unintended consequences like overeating during the eating window.

Furthermore, while intermittent fasting can lead to weight loss through calorie restriction, it's important to acknowledge that any form of calorie restriction is likely to result in weight loss. The unique benefits of intermittent fasting, such as neuroprotection and anti-inflammatory effects, while promising, still require more comprehensive, long-term research to be fully understood.

The Need to Purchase the Program

Access to the Galveston Diet program is not free. Depending on the level of engagement you choose, it can cost anywhere from $59 to $199. While this fee provides you with valuable resources such as curriculum, meal plans, recipes, and educational materials, it may present a financial barrier to some individuals.

Not everyone is willing or able to invest in a paid program for weight loss, particularly when there are free or lower-cost dieting alternatives available. This aspect of the Galveston Diet may limit its accessibility to women who would benefit from its principles but cannot afford the program's cost.

Real-Life Experiences with the Galveston Diet

To provide a well-rounded view of the Galveston Diet, it's essential to hear from individuals who have tried the program. Many women have shared their experiences, both positive and negative, with this diet.

Real-Life Success Stories

Several women in perimenopause have reported success with the Galveston Diet. They attribute their weight loss and improved well-being to the diet's focus on anti-inflammatory foods and intermittent fasting. Some key takeaways from these success stories include:

- **Sustainable Weight Loss**: Many women have praised the Galveston Diet for its sustainability. They appreciate that it doesn't involve extreme restrictions and allows them to enjoy a variety of whole, nutritious foods. This approach has helped them maintain their weight loss over time.

- **Improved Hormonal Balance**: Some women have reported a reduction in perimenopausal symptoms, such as hot flashes and mood swings, after following the Galveston Diet. They credit the diet's focus on hormone-regulating foods for these positive changes.

- **Enhanced Overall Health**: Beyond weight loss, some individuals have noted improvements in their overall health. They report feeling more energetic, experiencing better sleep, and having clearer skin as a result of the diet's emphasis on whole foods.

Challenges and Drawbacks

While there are success stories, it's important to acknowledge the challenges and drawbacks experienced by some women on the Galveston Diet:

- **Difficulty with Intermittent Fasting**: Not everyone finds intermittent fasting easy to incorporate into their lives. Some women have struggled with the 16:8 fasting window, finding it challenging to abstain from food for 16 hours. This can lead to frustration and may not be a suitable approach for everyone.

- **Financial Considerations**: The cost of the Galveston Diet program has been a limitation for some. Women on a tight budget or those who are not comfortable investing in a paid program may be discouraged from trying the diet.

- **Lack of Quick Fixes**: The Galveston Diet does not promise instant or miraculous results. While this is a positive aspect in terms of sustainability, it may not appeal to those seeking rapid weight loss solutions.

Chapter 7:
Is the Galveston Diet Right for You?

Perimenopausal women often find themselves in the midst of significant physical and hormonal changes that can lead to frustrating weight gain. The Galveston Diet offers a promising solution, but it's essential to determine if this approach is the right fit for your individual circumstances. In this chapter, we will delve into the critical considerations, alternative approaches to hormonal balance and weight loss, and expert opinions to help you make an informed decision about whether the Galveston Diet aligns with your health goals and needs.

Consideration of Individual Factors: Health Conditions, Dietary Preferences, and Lifestyle

Health Conditions

Before embarking on any dietary journey, it's crucial to assess your overall health and the presence of any medical conditions. Perimenopausal women can have a range of health concerns, such as diabetes, hypertension, or thyroid disorders. Here's how to navigate these considerations:

1. Diabetes: If you have diabetes or prediabetes, it's essential to consult with your healthcare provider before starting the Galveston Diet. While the diet emphasizes anti-inflammatory foods and intermittent fasting, these components can affect blood sugar levels. Your doctor can provide guidance on managing your condition while following the diet.

2. Hypertension: High blood pressure is another common health issue in perimenopausal women. The Galveston Diet's focus on whole, unprocessed foods can be beneficial, as it reduces sodium intake and encourages a heart-healthy lifestyle. However, again, it's advisable to consult with a healthcare provider for personalized recommendations.

3. Thyroid Disorders: Women often experience thyroid imbalances during menopause. The Galveston Diet's emphasis on anti-inflammatory foods can support thyroid health. However, it's essential to monitor your thyroid levels and discuss any dietary changes with your endocrinologist.

Dietary Preferences

Dietary preferences vary greatly among individuals, and the Galveston Diet may or may not align with your food choices. Here are some considerations:

1. Vegetarian or Vegan: If you follow a vegetarian or vegan diet, you can adapt the Galveston Diet to meet your preferences. While the diet promotes lean proteins like fish and poultry, you can find plant-based alternatives rich in protein, such as tofu, legumes, and quinoa.

2. Gluten-Free: The Galveston Diet's focus on whole foods is compatible with a gluten-free lifestyle. Whole grains like rice, quinoa, and oats can replace gluten-containing grains.

3. Food Allergies: If you have food allergies or sensitivities, you can adjust the diet to exclude problematic foods while still maintaining its core principles.

Lifestyle

Your daily routines, work obligations, and family life can greatly influence your ability to follow a specific diet. Consider these lifestyle factors:

1. Work Schedule: If your work schedule involves irregular hours or frequent travel, intermittent fasting may be challenging. You can explore flexible fasting schedules that align with your lifestyle.

2. Family and Social Life: Family gatherings, social events, and dining out with friends may pose challenges while following a structured diet. It's crucial to find strategies for maintaining your dietary goals within the context of your social life.

3. Exercise Routine: The Galveston Diet complements a healthy exercise routine. Consider how your workout schedule fits into the diet plan and how it may need adjustment.

Alternative Approaches to Hormonal Balance and Weight Loss for Perimenopausal Women

While the Galveston Diet offers a unique approach to weight loss for perimenopausal women, there are alternative strategies worth exploring. These approaches take into account hormonal balance and overall well-being:

1. Mediterranean Diet: The Mediterranean diet is known for its heart-healthy and anti-inflammatory components. It emphasizes fruits, vegetables, whole grains, lean protein, and healthy fats, making it a suitable alternative to the

Galveston Diet. Additionally, the Mediterranean diet allows for a more flexible approach to intermittent fasting.

2. Low-Carb Diet: Some women find success in managing their weight through a low-carb diet. Reducing carbohydrate intake can help regulate blood sugar and minimize insulin spikes, addressing one of the key concerns in perimenopausal weight gain.

3. Mindful Eating: Rather than following a specific diet plan, some women prefer to adopt a mindful eating approach. This focuses on listening to your body's hunger and fullness cues, making healthier food choices, and maintaining a balanced diet without strict rules.

4. Traditional Weight Loss Programs: Conventional weight loss programs that emphasize calorie control and regular exercise can be effective for perimenopausal women. While they may not specifically address hormonal balance, these programs can lead to sustainable weight loss.

Expert Opinions and Recommendations on Choosing the Right Diet Plan

It's always advisable to seek guidance from healthcare professionals and registered dietitians when making decisions about your dietary and weight management strategies. Here are some expert opinions and recommendations to consider:

1. Consult a Registered Dietitian: A registered dietitian can assess your individual health status, dietary preferences, and lifestyle and provide personalized recommendations. They can help you tailor the Galveston Diet or explore alternative approaches.

2. Healthcare Provider's Input: Your primary care physician or a specialist can offer insight into how the Galveston Diet may impact your specific health conditions. They can also monitor your progress and make necessary adjustments.

3. Evaluate Your Goals: Consider your weight loss and health goals. Are you primarily focused on weight loss, or are you equally concerned about improving your overall health and well-being? Different diets may align with different objectives.

4. Experiment and Monitor: Regardless of the diet you choose, it's essential to monitor your progress. Track your weight, energy levels, mood, and overall health. If you don't see the desired results, be open to adjusting your approach.

Chapter 8:
Tips for Success on the Galveston Diet

In Chapter 8, we'll delve into the essential aspects of success on the Galveston Diet. We'll explore practical tips for staying motivated and consistent with the diet, strategies for overcoming challenges and setbacks, and guidance on maintaining a healthy relationship with food while following this unique dietary plan.

Practical Tips for Staying Motivated and Consistent with the Diet

Staying motivated and consistent with any diet plan is crucial for achieving your weight loss and health goals. The Galveston Diet, with its focus on anti-inflammatory foods and intermittent fasting, is no exception. Here are some practical tips to help you stay on track:

1. **Set Clear Goals:** Before starting the Galveston Diet, define your specific weight loss or health improvement goals. Having a clear target will keep you motivated and accountable.

2. **Track Your Progress:** Keep a journal of your meals, fasting periods, and any changes in your body, such as weight, energy levels, or mood. Tracking your progress can help you see the positive effects of the diet over time.

3. **Find an Accountability Partner:** Sharing your journey with a friend or family member can provide extra motivation and support. You can exchange experiences, recipes, and successes to stay on course together.

4. **Celebrate Small Wins:** Celebrate your achievements, no matter how small they may seem. Whether it's losing a few pounds or resisting the temptation of processed foods, acknowledging your progress can boost your motivation.

5. **Plan Your Meals:** Meal planning can help you stay consistent by ensuring you have the right foods available. Prepare your meals in advance and have healthy snacks on hand to avoid making impulsive, unhealthy choices.

6. **Variety is Key:** Experiment with different recipes and foods to keep your meals exciting. Variety prevents boredom and makes it easier to stick with the diet.

7. **Stay Informed:** Educate yourself about the Galveston Diet and its principles. Knowing why you're following a certain eating pattern can strengthen your commitment.

8. **Seek Supportive Communities:** Join online forums, social media groups, or local meet-up groups dedicated to the Galveston Diet. Sharing experiences with like-minded individuals can provide encouragement and valuable insights.

Strategies for Overcoming Challenges and Setbacks

Challenges and setbacks are inevitable when embarking on any diet. It's important to recognize these obstacles and have strategies in place to overcome them. Here's how to navigate common hurdles:

1. **Cravings and Temptations:** You may occasionally crave processed foods or sugary snacks. To combat this, have healthy alternatives readily available. For

instance, choose whole fruit or nuts when cravings
strike.

2. **Social Pressure:** Social gatherings or family events
   can be tricky when following a specific diet.
   Communicate your dietary restrictions to friends
   and family in advance. Alternatively, offer to bring a
   dish that aligns with the Galveston Diet to ensure
   there's something suitable for you.

3. **Plateaus:** Weight loss plateaus can be discouraging.
   Remember that plateaus are a normal part of the
   journey. Continue following the diet and consider
   adding more physical activity to break through the
   plateau.

4. **Lack of Time:** Many people find it challenging to
   cook nutritious meals due to busy schedules. Make
   use of meal prep and batch cooking to save time.
   Cook large portions and freeze individual servings
   for convenience.

5. **Travel and Dining Out:** When traveling or dining out,
   research restaurant menus in advance and choose
   dishes that align with the Galveston Diet. You can

also pack healthy snacks to avoid unhealthy choices during transit.

6. **Boredom with Food:** Some individuals get bored with the same meals. Combat food monotony by trying new recipes, experimenting with different spices, or seeking inspiration from fellow Galveston dieters.

7. **Health Hiccups:** If you encounter health issues or side effects, consult a healthcare professional promptly. Do not hesitate to modify the diet under professional guidance.

8. **Stay Patient:** Understand that changes may not happen overnight. Weight loss and health improvements take time. Patience is a virtue when following any dietary plan.

Guidance on Maintaining a Healthy Relationship with Food

A healthy relationship with food is integral to your overall well-being, especially when following a specific diet. Here's how to maintain a positive relationship with food while on the Galveston Diet:

1. **Avoid Food Guilt:** Don't punish yourself for occasional indulgences or deviations from the diet. Guilt can lead to emotional eating and derail your progress.

2. **Practice Mindful Eating:** Pay attention to your body's hunger and fullness cues. Eating mindfully helps prevent overeating and promotes a better understanding of your dietary needs.

3. **Listen to Your Cravings:** Occasionally, your body may signal specific cravings. Instead of suppressing them, find healthier ways to satisfy those cravings within the framework of the Galveston Diet. For example, opt for dark chocolate or fruit when you crave sweets.

4. **Enjoy Social Eating:** Don't let dietary restrictions isolate you from social events. Focus on the social aspect of dining, not just the food. Engage in conversations and activities to make mealtime enjoyable.

5. **Balance Your Diet:** Ensure you're meeting your nutritional needs. If you have concerns about your

nutrient intake, consult a registered dietitian or healthcare professional for guidance.

6. **Self-Compassion:** Be kind to yourself throughout your journey. Understand that perfection is not the goal; consistency and progress are what truly matter.

Chapter 9:
Enhancing Your Journey with Exercise, Stress Management, and Quality Sleep

In the pursuit of holistic well-being and effective weight management during the perimenopausal years, the Galveston Diet provides a strong foundation. However, to truly optimize your health and ensure the best outcomes, it is vital to understand and incorporate the critical elements that complement this dietary approach: exercise, stress management, and quality sleep. In this chapter, we will delve into each of these elements, exploring their significance and the ways in which they can enhance the benefits of the Galveston Diet.

Importance of Exercise and Physical Activity in Conjunction with the Galveston Diet

Exercise: A Vital Component for Perimenopausal Women

As perimenopausal women, our bodies undergo significant changes. Hormonal fluctuations, muscle loss, and changes in metabolism can lead to increased fat storage, especially around the abdominal area. This is where exercise comes into play.

Exercise is not just about shedding pounds; it is a catalyst for a healthier, more vibrant life. Here's how it complements the Galveston Diet:

Muscle Maintenance and Fat Loss

With age, muscle mass tends to decline. This can lead to a slower metabolism and increased fat storage. Regular exercise, including strength training, helps to preserve and build lean muscle, which in turn accelerates fat loss. By incorporating resistance exercises into your routine, you can enhance the metabolic benefits of the Galveston Diet.

Enhanced Hormonal Balance

Exercise triggers the release of endorphins, often referred to as "feel-good" hormones. These endorphins not only improve mood but also play a role in regulating hormones. Engaging in physical activity can help reduce the stress hormone cortisol, leading to better hormonal balance. Hormones like cortisol, when chronically elevated, can contribute to weight gain, particularly around the midsection.

Improved Cardiovascular Health

Perimenopausal women are at an increased risk of heart disease due to hormonal changes. Regular cardiovascular exercise, such as brisk walking, cycling, or swimming, can improve heart health, lower blood pressure, and reduce the risk of heart-related complications.

Joint Health and Flexibility

As we age, joint health becomes more crucial. Engaging in regular, weight-bearing exercise helps maintain joint flexibility and reduces the risk of osteoarthritis. It also supports overall mobility and balance, reducing the likelihood of falls and injuries.

Stress Reduction

Stress management is a key component of the Galveston Diet. Exercise is an effective stress buster. It stimulates the production of brain chemicals like serotonin and norepinephrine, which help regulate mood and reduce stress and anxiety. By incorporating exercise into your routine, you can maximize the stress-reducing benefits of the diet.

Creating an Exercise Routine That Works for You

The type of exercise you choose should align with your preferences and health status. Whether it's yoga, strength training, swimming, or dance, the key is consistency. Aim for at least 150 minutes of moderate-intensity aerobic activity or 75 minutes of vigorous-intensity aerobic activity per week, combined with muscle-strengthening activities on two or more days a week.

Start slowly, especially if you are new to exercise or have been inactive for a while. Consult with a healthcare professional or fitness expert to tailor an exercise plan that suits your needs and abilities. Remember, it's not about being the fastest or the strongest but about nurturing your body and embracing a more active, healthier lifestyle.

Stress Management Techniques and Their Impact on Hormonal Balance and Weight Loss

Understanding the Connection Between Stress and Weight Gain

Stress, both emotional and physical, is an inevitable part of life. However, perimenopausal women often face an increased burden of stress due to hormonal changes, personal responsibilities, and societal expectations. Unfortunately, chronic stress can wreak havoc on hormonal balance and contribute to weight gain. Here's how it works:

The Cortisol Connection

Cortisol, often referred to as the "stress hormone," is released in response to stress. In the short term, cortisol is beneficial, helping your body respond to stressful situations. However, when stress is chronic, cortisol levels remain elevated, leading to numerous adverse effects, including:

- Increased abdominal fat storage

- Elevated blood sugar levels

- Increased appetite, particularly for unhealthy, high-calorie foods

These effects not only make it harder to lose weight but also pose significant health risks.

Stress Management Techniques for Perimenopausal Women

Effectively managing stress is integral to hormonal balance and weight loss. Here are stress management techniques that can complement the Galveston Diet:

1. Mindfulness Meditation

Mindfulness meditation is a practice that involves focusing your attention on the present moment, without judgment. It can help reduce stress, improve mood, and enhance emotional well-being. By incorporating mindfulness into your daily routine, you can counteract the negative impact of stress on your hormones.

2. Yoga and Relaxation Techniques

Yoga combines physical postures, breathing exercises, and meditation. It has been shown to reduce cortisol levels and promote relaxation. Even if you're not a seasoned yogi, basic yoga and relaxation techniques can be highly effective in managing stress.

3. Deep Breathing and Progressive Muscle Relaxation

Deep breathing exercises and progressive muscle relaxation techniques are simple yet powerful tools to alleviate stress. They help calm the mind and relax the body, reducing cortisol levels and promoting hormonal balance.

4. Time Management and Prioritization

Stress often arises from feeling overwhelmed by numerous responsibilities. Learning effective time management and prioritization strategies can help you regain control of your life and reduce stress levels.

5. Seeking Support and Professional Guidance

Don't hesitate to seek support from friends, family, or mental health professionals. Talking about your stressors and concerns can be therapeutic and provide valuable insights into managing stress effectively.

The Connection Between Stress Management and Weight Loss

By implementing stress management techniques, you not only promote hormonal balance but also create a more supportive environment for weight loss. Reducing cortisol levels can lead to a decrease in abdominal fat and better appetite control, making it easier to adhere to the Galveston Diet and achieve your desired weight loss goals.

Sleep and Its Role in the Overall Well-Being of Perimenopausal Women

The Perimenopausal Sleep Challenge

Quality sleep is an essential but often overlooked factor in weight management and overall well-being, particularly for perimenopausal women. During this life stage, sleep disturbances are common due to hormonal fluctuations, hot flashes, and night sweats. These issues can lead to chronic sleep deprivation and its associated consequences.

The Impact of Sleep on Hormonal Balance and Weight

The quality and duration of your sleep directly affect hormone regulation, including insulin, ghrelin (a hormone that stimulates appetite), and leptin (a hormone that regulates fullness). Sleep deprivation disrupts the balance of these hormones, making it more challenging to manage weight effectively. Here's how:

Insulin Resistance

Chronic sleep deprivation can lead to insulin resistance, a condition in which your cells don't respond effectively to insulin. This results in higher blood sugar levels, increased fat storage, and a greater risk of obesity and type 2 diabetes.

Increased Appetite

Inadequate sleep can disrupt the balance of ghrelin and leptin, leading to increased appetite and poor appetite control. This can result in overeating and a preference for high-calorie, unhealthy foods.

Hormonal Fluctuations

Sleep is critical for regulating hormones, including those that influence appetite and metabolism. Lack of sleep can lead to hormonal imbalances that hinder weight loss.

Stress Amplification

Poor sleep can exacerbate stress levels, increasing cortisol production. Elevated cortisol, as mentioned earlier, contributes to abdominal fat storage and weight gain.

Prioritizing Quality Sleep for Well-Being and Weight Management

Given the significant impact of sleep on hormonal balance and weight, it is crucial to prioritize quality sleep. Here are strategies to help you achieve a restful night:

1. Sleep Hygiene

Create a sleep-conducive environment by keeping your bedroom dark, quiet, and at a comfortable temperature. Remove electronic devices that emit blue light and disrupt circadian rhythms.

2. Consistent Sleep Schedule

Maintain a regular sleep schedule by going to bed and waking up at the same time each day, even on weekends. This helps regulate your body's internal clock.

3. Relaxation Techniques

Engage in relaxation practices before bedtime, such as reading, gentle stretching, or taking a warm bath. These activities can help signal to your body that it's time to wind down.

4. Limit Caffeine and Alcohol

Reduce or eliminate caffeine and alcohol consumption, especially in the hours leading up to bedtime. Both substances can interfere with sleep quality.

5. Seek Medical Advice

If sleep disturbances persist, consult with a healthcare professional or sleep specialist. They can diagnose and address any underlying sleep disorders.

Chapter 10:
Making Informed Decisions About Your Health

As you've journeyed through the pages of this ebook, you've gained a deep understanding of the Galveston Diet and how it addresses the challenges of perimenopausal weight gain. You've learned about the science behind this diet, its pros and cons, and whether it might be the right choice for you. Now, as we conclude this guide, we turn our attention to empowering you to make informed decisions about your health, and we stress the importance of consulting healthcare professionals and registered dietitians for personalized guidance. Additionally, we provide you with a wealth of resources and references for further reading, research, and support.

Empowering Readers to Make Informed Choices About Their Diet and Lifestyle

Empowerment begins with knowledge. Armed with information about the Galveston Diet, you're now better equipped to make decisions about your diet and lifestyle. Here are some key points to consider:

1. Understand Your Unique Needs

No one knows your body better than you do. Pay close attention to how your body responds to the Galveston Diet. Monitor your energy levels, mood, and any changes in weight. This self-awareness can help you adjust the diet to suit your individual needs.

2. Listen to Your Body

Your body is constantly sending signals about what it needs. Learn to listen to these signals. If you're hungry, eat. If you're full, stop. Pay attention to cravings and consider what they might indicate. Craving chocolate could be a sign of a magnesium deficiency, for example.

3. Set Realistic Goals

The Galveston Diet, like any other diet, is not a magic solution. It's a tool that can help you reach your goals. Be realistic about what you can achieve and in what time frame. Setting achievable goals will keep you motivated and prevent disappointment.

4. Stay Informed

The field of nutrition and health is continually evolving. Stay informed about the latest research and developments. Be open to adapting your diet and lifestyle based on new information. This might mean adjusting your approach or trying something new.

5. Consistency Is Key

No matter which diet you choose, consistency is essential. Even the most well-designed diet won't work if you only follow it sporadically. Stick to your chosen plan and monitor your progress regularly.

6. Seek Support

Surround yourself with a supportive community. Whether it's friends, family, or online groups, having a support system can make your journey towards a healthier lifestyle much more manageable. Share your experiences, challenges, and triumphs with those who understand and encourage your goals.

Encouragement to Consult Healthcare Professionals and Registered Dietitians for Personalized Guidance

While the Galveston Diet can be a valuable tool for perimenopausal women, it's crucial to remember that one size does not fit all. Your health is a complex interplay of genetics, lifestyle, and individual circumstances. Therefore, seeking personalized guidance from healthcare professionals and registered dietitians is strongly encouraged:

1. Consult Your Healthcare Provider

Before making any significant dietary changes, it's wise to consult your healthcare provider, especially if you have underlying health conditions or are taking medications. They can help ensure that your chosen diet plan is safe and appropriate for you.

2. Registered Dietitian Guidance

Registered dietitians are experts in nutrition and can provide you with tailored advice based on your specific needs. They can help you design a personalized diet plan that aligns with the principles of the Galveston Diet while addressing your unique dietary requirements.

3. Hormone and Health Assessment

A healthcare provider or endocrinologist can assess your hormone levels and overall health, helping you understand how hormonal changes during perimenopause may affect your weight and overall well-being. Based on these assessments, they can recommend appropriate interventions.

4. Blood Tests and Monitoring

Regular blood tests can provide critical insights into your health. These tests can help you and your healthcare provider track your progress, making necessary adjustments to your diet and lifestyle along the way.

5. Medication Management

If you have health conditions requiring medication, discuss the compatibility of your medication with your chosen diet. Adjustments may be needed, and your healthcare provider can guide you on the best approach.

6. Emotional and Psychological Support

Don't neglect the psychological aspect of your health journey. The emotional and psychological support from therapists or counselors can be invaluable, especially if you have a history of disordered eating or emotional eating patterns.

Resources and References for Further Reading, Research, and Support

Knowledge is power, and you have access to a vast array of resources to support your journey toward a healthier, happier you. Here are some suggestions for further reading, research, and support:

1. Books and Scientific Literature

- Explore books on nutrition, perimenopausal health, and weight management. Look for authoritative sources and scientific literature to deepen your understanding of the Galveston Diet and related topics.

2. Online Communities

- Join online communities, forums, or social media groups dedicated to perimenopausal health and weight management. Engage with others who share your experiences and seek advice and support.

3. Professional Organizations

- Connect with professional organizations such as the Academy of Nutrition and Dietetics to access reliable information and locate registered dietitians in your area.

4. Trusted Websites and Journals

- Explore reputable websites and medical journals for the latest research and evidence-based information on nutrition, health, and perimenopausal issues.

5. Apps and Tools

- Consider using health and fitness apps that can help you track your dietary intake, physical activity, and monitor your progress.

6. Support Groups

- Seek out local or virtual support groups for perimenopausal women. Sharing your experiences and challenges with others who are on a similar journey can be immensely beneficial.

Conclusion: Empowering Your Journey to Health and Happiness

As you reach the conclusion of this ebook, you've embarked on a journey of discovery, empowerment, and transformation in the context of the Galveston Diet. You've delved into the intricacies of perimenopausal weight gain, explored the science behind the Galveston Diet, weighed its pros and cons, and learned how to make informed decisions about your health and well-being. Now, it's time to reflect on your newfound knowledge and chart the course ahead.

The Power of Knowledge

Knowledge is the cornerstone of your journey. The insights you've gained about the Galveston Diet and perimenopausal health are invaluable. You now understand how hormonal changes, lifestyle factors, and the Galveston Diet intersect to influence your well-being. Armed with this knowledge, you are better equipped to make informed choices about your diet and lifestyle.

Understanding your unique needs, listening to your body, setting realistic goals, staying informed, being consistent, and seeking support are the pillars of empowerment. These principles are not confined to the Galveston Diet alone but extend to any path you choose in pursuit of health and happiness. Your journey is a personal one, and your decisions should reflect your individuality.

The Role of Healthcare Professionals and Registered Dietitians

While knowledge is a potent tool, expertise is indispensable. Healthcare professionals and registered dietitians are your trusted allies in this journey. Their guidance is instrumental in ensuring that your chosen dietary and lifestyle modifications are safe, effective, and tailored to your specific needs.

Consulting your healthcare provider and collaborating with a registered dietitian can help you navigate the complexities of health during perimenopause. They can conduct hormone and health assessments, monitor your progress, and make adjustments as needed. For those with underlying health conditions or those taking medications, their expertise ensures that your health remains a top priority.

Moreover, don't overlook the psychological and emotional aspects of your health journey. Therapists and counselors can provide invaluable support, especially if you have a history of emotional or disordered eating patterns. Your mental well-being is intertwined with your physical health, and addressing both aspects is vital.

Empowering and Adapting

Empowerment, as you've learned, extends far beyond your dietary choices. It is a mindset, a way of approaching your health with confidence and self-awareness. It is about recognizing that you have the power to shape your own path, to make choices that align with your goals and values.

Adaptation is also a critical component of your journey. The Galveston Diet, like any other, may require adjustments. It's crucial to remain open to new information, research, and evolving best practices in the field of nutrition and health. If something isn't working as expected, be willing to try a different approach or make necessary modifications.

The Resources at Your Fingertips

Your journey is not solitary; you have an array of resources at your fingertips. Books, scientific literature, online communities, professional organizations, trusted websites, journals, apps, and support groups are available to you. These resources can expand your knowledge, provide support, and connect you with like-minded individuals who share your experiences.

Consider this ebook as the starting point of a lifelong commitment to your health and happiness. Your journey does not end here; it continues to evolve and grow as you adapt to new information and circumstances.

Your Journey Towards Health and Happiness

In the end, your journey is about more than just losing weight; it's about reclaiming your health, vitality, and happiness. The Galveston Diet, with its focus on anti-inflammatory foods and intermittent fasting, is a promising tool for perimenopausal women. However, it's just one path among many.

You have the power to make choices that resonate with your values, preferences, and unique needs. Whether you choose the Galveston Diet or another approach, your journey is a testament to your commitment to a healthier and happier you.

Remember that your health journey is a lifelong adventure, and there is no one-size-fits-all solution. Seek guidance, stay informed, be adaptable, and embrace the support systems available to you. Your journey may have its ups and downs, but with each step, you move closer to a life filled with well-being, vitality, and contentment.

The chapters you've read and the knowledge you've gained serve as a compass for your path. The destination? A life where you are in control, where your health and happiness are your priorities, and where you thrive in the face of perimenopausal challenges.

Your journey has only just begun, and the future is brimming with possibilities. Let this be a celebration of your commitment to health and happiness, the first step in a remarkable adventure. Your health is your greatest treasure, and your happiness is your ultimate goal. Embrace your journey, trust in your choices, and savor every moment of your pursuit of health and happiness.